We think of breast
After all, there are appro
breast cancer on year-to-year basis. As physicians, we are concerned about the physical effects of breast cancer and its psychological impact. The physical impact includes the disfigurement caused by breast cancer surgery and the psychological impact includes the fear of dying from breast cancer as well as the alteration of body image and how it impacts on sexuality.

We do not think of breast cancer as a disease of men even though 5000 men come down with it on year-to-year basis. Men are supposed to be stoic. Loss of a breast shouldn't lead to physical disfigurement. Loss of the male breast shouldn't lead to alterations of body image and shouldn't impact sexuality. However, what women experience in dealing with breast cancer also applies to men. This book deals with one man's journey with male breast cancer. It is indeed eye-opening to read the impact of breast cancer as experienced by a man.

— **Dr. Jacob Bitran**
Head Oncologist of Oncology Specialists,
Lutheran General Cancer Care Center, Park Ridge, IL

Many people do not realize that breast cancer can occur in men. It is not common in men, but it is important for men to see their doctor right away if they notice a breast lump. The first step is to get a mammogram and an ultrasound. (Yes, a mammogram can be done on men!)

Men who may be at increased risk are those with a strong family history of breast cancer, those with previous radiation exposure, and those with high levels of estrogen (from diseases such as cirrhosis or Klinefelter's.) Breast cancer in men is very treatable and even curable if caught early.

— **Dr. Heidi Memmel M.D.**
Director Of Breast Surgery,
Caldwell Breast Center

I Have WHAT???

ONE MAN'S JOURNEY THROUGH BREAST CANCER

RICHARD W. WIENER

PUBLISHED BY FIDELI PUBLISHING INC.

I Have WHAT???

ONE MAN'S JOURNEY THROUGH BREAST CANCER

©Copyright 2012, Richard W. Wiener

All Rights Reserved.

No part of this book may be reproduced, stored in electronic format, or transmitted without written permission from the author.

ISBN: 978-1-60414-592-2

Fideli Publishing Inc.
119 W. Morgan St.
Martinsville, IN 46151

www.FideliPublishing.com

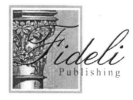

DEDICATION

This book is dedicated to all the men and women who have, or have had, breast cancer.

TABLE OF CONTENTS

Dedication 3
Foreword vii

CHAPTER 1
The Discovery 1

CHAPTER 2
The Surgery 4

CHAPTER 3
The Hospital Stay 6

CHAPTER 4
Home At Last 9

CHAPTER 5
The Oncologist 12

CHAPTER 6
The Port 15

CHAPTER 7
Week One 18

CHAPTER 8
Week Two 26

CHAPTER 9
Week Three 31

CHAPTER 10
Week Four 37

Photo Album 45

CHAPTER 11	
Week Five	51
CHAPTER 12	
Week Six	58
CHAPTER 13	
Week Seven	64
CHAPTER 14	
Week Eight	71
CHAPTER 15	
Week Nine	78
CHAPTER 16	
Week Ten	84
CHAPTER 17	
Week Eleven	90
CHAPTER 18	
Week Twelve	98
About the Author	106

FOREWORD

"You have to be kidding me! Impossible! Must be some kind of mistake! Are you positive? I have what???"

This is the story of my experience with breast cancer, from the discovery of a lump in my breast through my chemotherapy treatments. It includes everything I went through to increase my odds for survival.

Everything you will read is pure fact, written during the course of my treatment. If I can save one man's life, then it will be well worth it.

CHAPTER 1

THE DISCOVERY

On February 9, 2012, I made a discovery that would change my life forever. While showering, I found a rather hard lump by the nipple of my left breast. I realize that most men would have dismissed, it but not me. I've always been very proactive about my health. I just had to have this thing checked out.

The next morning, I made an appointment to have my internist take a look. He felt the lump and measured it. Then he sent me to a breast surgeon for a better look. My physician told me that the odds were in my favor, as only one in every hundred breast cancers were found in men. He continued to tell me that, if it was cancer, then I had caught it early and it would be treated.

So on February 20, I went to see the breast surgeon. Before she would see me, I had to go through a mammogram on both breasts, and then an ultrasound on my left one. I was sure the ultrasound would find the lump that I was feeling. Actually, you could not miss it.

I was then led into another room, where I patiently waited for the doctor. My wait was not long, as the doctor walked in and we had a brief conversation about how I had found my lump, as most men do not check themselves.

She then pulled up the results of my two tests on the computer. They did show a tumor, which was 1.4 centimeters in diameter. She told me that was small, and she wanted to do a biopsy. Never one to put things off, I asked if it could be done right away.

I wish I could tell you that the biopsy was not painful, but that would be a lie. The needle that was stuck in me looked ten inches long. Four slices of the tumor were removed, and I was told that the doctor would call me the next day with the results.

I always think the worst but hope for the best. I was sitting on my couch at home when the phone rang. It was the doctor, who had reviewed the pathology report from my biopsy. I jokingly asked her if I should be seated — and she said yes. Now my stomach was in my mouth. She told me that I had breast cancer, but that the tumor was small. Men usually do not find it until it's already 2.5 centimeters. She told me that I was at grade one, and that I should come in to discuss the options.

As soon as I hung up, I put in a call to my late wife's oncologist. My wife had passed away from breast cancer five years earlier, and I knew her oncologist well. I felt he was very good, and I trusted him with my life. He was shocked to hear from me. After I told him what was happening, he said I had no other option but to remove my left breast. After that, he said, I should come see him and we would discuss further treatment.

I saw the surgeon on February 24. I told her that I had spoken with my oncologist, and he had recommended a simple mastectomy. I went on to tell her that I wanted this shit out of my body as soon as possible. With that said, we scheduled my surgery for February 28. At the time, everything seemed surreal to me. Waiting was not an option.

CHAPTER 2

THE SURGERY

I find it amazing how things are done today. Instead of checking into the hospital the night before, I was told to check in at noon for a surgery scheduled at 2 p.m.

My daughter picked me up at 11:30 a.m., and we left for the hospital. I was not even nervous, which surprised me. I always say, "it is what it is, and just face it." No one gets through this life unscathed.

We arrived right on time and I checked into nuclear medicine, which was my first stop. This stop was not very pleasant. Before doing a mastectomy, the doctor would shoot dye into me, which would travel to the closest lymph nodes. This would tell the doctor which lymph nodes to take out and biopsy. The nodes would be immediately sent to pathology and, if any of those come back positive for a tumor, then more lymph nodes would be taken out. What the doctor wanted to see were clear margins, showing the cancer did not advance.

So off I went, wheeled into a room that looked like the operating room on "Grey's Anatomy." What was done next still makes me cringe when I think about it. The dye was shot in four times, in the nipple. I was numbed, but I could still feel it—and I mean feel it. I had a high pain threshold but, as I'd gotten older, my tolerance had gotten much lower. I had endured quite a bit of pain in my sixty-six years.

Now I was ready for surgery. Before heading into the operating room, the surgeon came in to talk with me about the procedure. She wanted me to know everything that was going on. She drew an outline on my soon-to-be-gone left breast. Now I was ready— as ready as I could ever be. It had been about twenty years since my knee surgery, but I kind of knew what to expect.

The operating room could be quite intimidating. Actually scary. As soon as I was wheeled in on a cart, I asked for the drugs. After that, I do not remember anything until I woke up in recovery. I was quite groggy when the surgeon came in and told me that some tumor was found in two nodes, and that she'd removed fifteen. That put me in stage two. She also told me that I had a surgical drain that I would wear for about ten days. But two words she told me forever embedded in my mind: "treatable" and "curable."

CHAPTER 3

THE HOSPITAL STAY

When I came to after surgery, everything was still fuzzy. I was in recovery, and didn't even remember being carted into my room. It was around 6:30 p.m., my daughter was there, and I had a private room.

I wasn't feeling any pain, probably because of the pain medication. I was a little nauseous, but I was given anti-nausea meds through my IV bag. I do remember the nurse asking me if I was hungry, as the kitchen was about to close.

My daughter ordered me a hamburger and some mac and cheese, just in case I got hungry later on. Food was the last thing on my mind. I did want something to drink, though, as my throat was a little raw from the tube they must have put down me. Thank the lord for anesthesia.

The nurse came into my room and showed me my drain, which kind of freaked me out. I am actually quite squeamish when it comes to things like this. The nurse also said that, if I could pee, she could release me to go home. Feeling the way I did, though, there was no reason for me to go home. I was lightheaded and wanted to just rest.

I kind of lost all sensation of time. I asked the nurse for more anti-nausea meds. At the same time, my dinner arrived. I took one bite of the hamburger, and had to look at it, as I thought that they'd replaced it with a hockey puck. Yuck! Then I tried the mac and cheese, and *that* was horrible. Yuck again.

I sent my daughter home, as she had to drive an hour to get home and I just wanted to rest. I also wanted to pee. You see, the hospital never lets you go home until your body starts working again. When you are put out, your body goes to sleep with you.

It must have been around 1:30 a.m. when I opened my eyes and was starting to feel better. I was actually hungry. A good friend of mine had brought me a bagel earlier in the evening. I grabbed it and made short work of it.

The trouble with hospitals was that, when you finally got to sleep, someone was in your room checking your vitals. So much for sleeping. I asked the nurse to unhook me from the IV so I could walk around. It felt good to get off the bed and get on my own two feet. I even attempted to pee again, with no results.

At about 9 a.m., my surgeon and my primary physician came in the room together. My surgeon told me again that two lymph nodes had some tumor and that she removed fifteen nodes altogether, and that was why I needed the drain. She told me that I would need to keep the drain until I drained less than 30 cc (cubic centimeters) of fluid per 24-hour period. She told me that, before I got discharged, I would be shown how to manage the drain. My primary physician ordered me some Flomax to help me pee. Thank the lord, as it did not take long after my first pill for me to start peeing.

Around 5 p.m. I was told that I could go home. I was also told that a mobile nurse would be calling me to set up a schedule for her to come to my home and change my dressing. I was a little worried about that, as there was no way I could change the bandages myself.

My chariot arrived around 6 p.m., and I had to wait for a wheelchair to ride me out; it was hospital policy that you must be wheeled out. My nurse went over my discharge papers, and gave me a script for a painkiller.

So on the way home, we made a stop to fill the prescription and pick up some groceries. All the while, I was thinking something must be wrong because I'd just had surgery, and I was feeling great.

CHAPTER 4

HOME AT LAST

It sure was good to be home. It felt even better to know that my mobile nurse would be coming over every other day to change the dressing, which included an ace bandage wrapped around my chest. Squeamish me even checked and emptied the fluid from my drain every twelve hours.

Sleeping was not easy at this point. I am a sleeper who rolls from my back to my stomach and back to my back. The drain made that a little uncomfortable. The spot that I found to give me my best sleep was the couch in my man cave. There I couldn't roll, or I would end up on the floor.

The first few times the nurse came to change my bandages, I could not make myself look at my scar. It was toward the end of the week before I actually glanced down to see how I looked.

To my surprise, it did not look bad. For a woman, I am sure it is more devastating. I was asked if I wanted reconstructive surgery, and I kind of laughed. More surgery was not in my plans, especially at my age. I am a little self-conscious, so I would just wear a t-shirt when I hit the pool in Las Vegas.

Every twelve hours, I measured the drainage from my drain. It was slowing down, and was at 40 cc for a 24-hour period. I could not wait until it slowed to 30 cc, so I could get this thing removed. I had already set up my post-op appointment with the surgeon who would remove the drain. I was hoping that I could go in earlier, but that didn't look like the case. I also made an appointment with my oncologist for a few days after the drain would be removed.

I had a history with my oncologist, as he had also been my wife's oncologist. She had passed away in 2007 from breast cancer, so I was quite knowledgeable about it. I also did quite a bit of reading and knew what to expect in the way of treatment, so I would not be surprised.

Monday, March 12, was my post-op to have the drain removed. Funny to say, but I did not let the drain hinder me in what I did during the thirteen days it was in. I went to hockey games, to movies, and out to dinner. As long as I felt good, I did what I wanted.

The drain removal was one of the easier things done to me in the last two weeks. It took about one minute for the surgeon to take it out. She also removed the bandage and told me that the narrow strips over my incision would come off in time. I could now shower the right way. Previously, I had to improvise so I could wash my hair without exposing my incision to the shower water.

With that done, I was now ready for the next stage, which was my visit to the oncologist. My appointment was on Thursday, March 15. I really wanted to get in and get started on my treatment.

The nurse came one last time to release me from her care, and had me sign more papers. Since the beginning of this process, I'd signed more papers than I would for the closing on my house.

I knew that when I saw the doctor on Thursday, he would put me through chemotherapy. After what I had witnessed with my wife's treatment, I knew that I was in for a grueling time. My attitude was, "let's bring it on."

CHAPTER 5

THE ONCOLOGIST

This was starting to blow my mind. I never thought I would say that I had an oncologist.

I did a lot of reading on WebMD about whatever ailed me, and tried to be as informed as I possibly could. I knew that I would have to have chemotherapy, and I also knew that everyone's body reacts differently to the side effects. The thought of losing my hair was driving me crazy. I'd had a full head of hair all my life, which would make this hard on me. But then again, I was assured that it would grow back. I remember, when I was young, I told my mother that I did not care if my hair turned orange, as long as I had it. The other thing that I hoped could be controlled was the nausea. I hate to puke!

I did not have to wait long for the doctor to see me. He was shocked when, over the phone, I had told him about what I had. At least there was some comfort in not having to go to a stranger.

I asked him if he'd reviewed my pathology report, which he had. He told me that I did catch it early, and that it was treatable and curable. My two favorite words.

He then proceeded to tell me that if we did absolutely nothing, I would have a 65 percent survival rate for five years. If we did chemo, the survival rate went up to 89 percent for five years. Then 95 percent for seven years and 100 percent for ten years. After the chemo, I would be on Tamoxifen for five years.

This was a no-brainer to me. I was playing the odds. I was hoping that my luck was better than my having one of the 1 percent of breast cancer cases affecting men. He went on to tell me that I would lose my hair and feel fatigued. I could deal with that, but I knew from my reading that there were many other side effects that might hit me.

I would be assigned a nurse, who would be my resource for the chemo. My doctor told me that I would have four rounds of chemo, one every three weeks. My first one would be on March 30, and the last on May 31. He also suggested that I have a port put in, as chemo is hard on the veins and the port would make it easier for me. Because I had my surgery on February 28, I would not be starting the treatments until a month after, which would give me time to have the port put in and to heal before I got started.

This all felt surreal to me, but I am a person who does not procrastinate and wants things done in a rather quick manner. So as soon as I got home, I called my nurse to touch base with her. We had a nice conversation, and she set up my appointment to have the port put in my right arm on March 20. Since I would be in la la land, I needed a ride. So I asked a very good friend of mine to drive me and, of course, he said he would.

I hated asking people for favors, but I had no choice and did not want to take a cab. So I arranged the time to be picked up, allowing for traffic, as I did not want to be late.

I love the summer and always look forward to it. But now, I just wanted it to be August already. By then, hopefully, I would be back to myself once more.

CHAPTER 6

THE PORT

I must say that the only ports I thought I would ever see were off a cruise ship. Unfortunately, the next port would be in my right arm. I had two choices—in my arm or in my chest. I opted for the arm, as I did not want to have the circular item in my chest. Every time my blood was drawn or I was given an IV, it would be through the port.

It was now March 20, and my appointment was at 2 p.m. I was told to be at the hospital an hour beforehand, so I had my friend pick me up at 12:30 p.m. The trip to the hospital was like riding in a cab in New York with a driver from another country who did not grasp the art of driving here. I was constantly stepping on my imaginary brake, and the ride probably aged me another ten years. You see, I rarely let someone else drive me, as I am a very nervous passenger.

After parking the car, we walked into the hospital, headed for the radiation reception area, and checked in. I did not have to wait very long, as they were ready for me. I was asked my name and date of birth eight times, I guess in order to avoid a mistake.

Once I'd proven I was not an imposter, I was given a gown and told to undress from the waist up and lie down on the bed. The nurses were extremely nice and explained the whole procedure to me. Then the doctor who would be putting in the port came in. He also explained what would happen and asked if I had any questions. I was somewhat familiar with this process, as my wife had a port put in at the same place.

I was then wheeled into a room that looked like an operating room, which it probably was. It had these big, intimidating machines, which helped the doctor guide the port into my vein. I had to slide onto a narrow table, and an IV was put in for what I called the "happy drugs." Before I knew it, the procedure was over and I was wheeled back to my area to clear my head from the drugs. You gotta love those happy drugs.

I was really hungry, as I'd had nothing to eat for more than fifteen hours. They brought me some water and some Lorna Doones. Those cookies tasted great, and I devoured them in seconds. My head was pretty clear now, and I was ready to get out of dodge.

Before I left, the nurse came in with discharge directions for me and some supplies to take home. I had three stitches in my arm that would have to stay in for ten days. This would coincide with my first chemo appointment. I had to change the bandage every day, and could not get the stitches wet. To take a shower, I had to find a way to cover them. The nurse advised me to take the plastic sleeve from my daily paper, put it on my arm, and tape the ends so water would not penetrate. That sounded easy enough. I was sent home with enough supplies to last until my appointment in ten days.

I was ready to run out of there, but hospital procedure required for me to be wheeled out in a wheelchair. After I blew kisses to all the young, good-looking nurses, I headed in my chariot to the front door, where I waited for my friend to bring up the car for my frightening journey home.

My friends asked all the time if I was nervous about this bump in my road, as I seemed so calm. To tell you the truth, I did appear calm on the outside, but my main worry was the side effects of the chemo. I saw what chemo did to my wife, and it was very hard to watch. I knew that everyone reacted differently, and that her cancer was advanced while mine was not, and I am a strong individual. Another concern was that I lived alone, so there was no one around if I experienced a problem. I had friends who offered to stay with me if it got bad and, even though I am stubborn, I thought I might take them up on it.

Now I was just waiting for March 30 so I could begin my treatment. I just had to remember that I would get better and eventually be back to my old, lovable self.

CHAPTER 7

WEEK ONE

I got absolutely zero sleep the night before my first treatment. While I did read a lot to have some knowledge on what to expect, I was still heading into uncharted waters with this. My main concern was the side effects. I did know that some people who had jobs didn't miss much time during chemo. Fortunately, I was already retired, so I did not have to worry about that.

My first chemo appointment was at 11 a.m. My daughter-in-law would be taking me each time, and would stay with me for the four chemo sessions. I do realize how lucky I was to have her. She had meals for me to put in my freezer, and questions for my nurse. I wouldn't think of having my daughter come with me, because she was six months pregnant and in a new job, and I did not want her taking time off work.

I got to the lab, which was on the first floor of the brand-new cancer center, to have my blood drawn. That would be the first thing done on every visit. The blood had to be drawn from my hand, as I could not have it done in the arm because of the port. I had so many needles in me that I was starting to feel like a pincushion.

After my blood was drawn, I headed up to oncology, on the second floor. I checked in and waited for my chemo nurse. I hated just sitting and waiting. I was actually counting the days until I could start my treatment. The faster I started it, the sooner I would get done.

Once I was called in, the first thing the technicians did was get my weight and height so, they could figure a formula to tell them what my dose of chemo would be. Everyone is different, and their dosage depends on the formula. Losing weight or gaining weight would change the dosage.

Next we were led into my private cubicle, which had a recliner for me, a chair for my guest, and a TV to watch if so desired. My daughter-in-law and I settled in and waited to meet the nurse who was assigned to me.

We did not have to wait long before she came in with a folder to educate me on what would happen. The first thing she did was access my port. It hurt for a mega second, but I was used to it. She started my anti-nausea drug, which would run for a half an hour before she started the major drugs. Being nauseous was one fear I had. She told me that I was given five days' worth of the drug, which should do the trick, and also gave me a prescription for pills that I would pick up on the way home, just in case I had any nausea after the five days.

We went over the possible side effects, what to do for them, and when to call if I experienced certain things. We set up my schedule of visits—March 30, April 19, May 19, and May 31. I also had to come in on April 12 to check my blood-cell count. Chemo lowers your white blood cell count, which lowers your resistance and makes you susceptible to infection. The part that would bother me was if my blood count made me delay the chemo and throw off my schedule.

I was given a list of meds and other things to get at the drugstore. I needed a digital thermometer to take my temperature, to make sure that I was not running a fever above 100.5 degrees. I also had to pick up vitamin B-6 to help with any neuropathy. Also on the list were Biodine mouthwash and toothpaste. I also picked up hand sanitizers for people to use when coming into my house, for fear of germs.

I was also told when to get my hair buzzed, which I scheduled for April 11. Hair, I was told, usually falls out on the seventeenth day or so. I was also told to continue going to the health club as long as I felt good, mainly because keeping your normal routine helps fight depression, which can be a major problem. Seeing that I could not sleep the previous night, I was given a prescription for a sleeping pill. I had never taken one before, but I did try one that first night. For what it's worth, I slept for three and a half hours, got up, and went back to bed for another three and a half hours.

Aching muscles and joints were also expected side effects. I could take Tylenol for that and, if it got bad enough, I had painkillers from my mastectomy that I'd never used.

The next day was Saturday, March 31, and I was having a good day. I took each day one at a time, waiting for the supposed side effects to hit, but I was ready for them. I drank sixty-four ounces of liquid a day to keep hydrated, which was a must. The part that would be really hard for me was feeling great one day and not great the next. I always kept in mind that everyone's body is different and handles medication in its own way. I was going to spend my day doing errands, then staying home to relax by watching basketball and hockey.

It was Monday, April 2, and I'd had a good weekend. I wanted to get up and hit the health club to do some walking, but today was much different than yesterday. I felt quite tired, and my legs were telling me to chill out. So instead of going for my anticipated long trip back to the club, I did a few errands and went out to breakfast with my morning paper as I usually did.

I knew that I had to take each day at a time and let my body dictate what I should do. I was drinking so much liquid that I kept peeing like a racehorse. One thing I did not want was to get dehydrated, which would be a major problem. Not being much of a water drinker, I chose to put Crystal Light lemonade in my water.

I was a little achy, but that was expected. All the while, I kept saying to myself, "I will get through this!" Tomorrow was another day.

Last night was not a good one. Even though I took a pill to help me relax, I was up at 3:30 a.m. Then back to bed, and I finally got up at 9 a.m. Not that I slept the whole time. I was experiencing aches in my ankles and knees like never before. I just could not find a comfortable spot for myself. This was day four of my first treatment. Two good and two bad.

Around 3 p.m. that afternoon, I had a sense of relief. The joint pain seemed to subside for a while. I just wanted a good night's sleep. I did know that I would not be able to sleep for long periods because of all the liquid I consumed during the day. Just call me Secretariat, as I sure peed like a horse.

I did something that day that I had not done before. I took a pain pill, hoping that it will take the edge off my aches. I also could not believe that I was going to get into bed to watch TV at 7:30 p.m., a record for me. The next day was Wednesday, April 4. Hopefully, a better day.

A good friend of mine who went through chemo told me that this stuff would mess with my sleep. Truer words were never spoken. After I actually got into bed at 7:30 p.m., I did fall asleep and, when I opened my eyes, it was 10:08 p.m. I decided to watch some TV and fell asleep again, this time getting up at midnight. I then decided to leave my bedroom and head for the basement to watch a movie.

I actually stayed there until 2 a.m., then headed back upstairs. I then fell asleep and awoke at 8:30 a.m. I was feeling a little better than the day before, as the aches in my ankles and knees seemed to disappear.

I was feeling well enough to take myself out to breakfast with the paper. This was a big accomplishment, considering the way I'd felt the last two days. It did feel good to get out of the house.

I spent an hour out of the house, then came back home to take a shower and shave, which made me feel better. I was hoping that I'd continue to feel better as the day went on. I just could not get over that tired feeling.

Sleep. What I would give for a good night's sleep. It was a good thing that I did not live in a small studio apartment, or I would have probably jumped out the window by that point. I did not get more than two hours of straight sleep. I kept changing rooms to find a comfortable spot. It also didn't help that I had a rather disturbing headache to go with my ankle and knee pains.

When I finally got up at 7:30 a.m., the day was rather long. Up early with nowhere to go. That morning I felt quite tired, and the headache had not left. I put in a call to my nurse for a painkiller prescription, something for my headache, and a sleeping pill. I will not medicate myself without an okay from my nurse.

The afternoon was better than the morning. I would take any improvement that I got. What pissed me off was that my nurse had not called me back yet, and it was close to 5 p.m. I was ready to go to the pharmacy to pick up my meds, but I had no idea if she called the script in. Another bad night, and my temper would be a little short. I had left two voicemails already. One thing about me is I never want to be a pest.

Seeing as I did feel better, I decided to take a five-minute ride to the pharmacy and ask if there was anything called in for me. Then back home to get into my position on the couch to watch my hockey game.

It was Thursday, April 5, and the next day was the end of the first week. All I could ask was that I'd get some rest that night. I don't pray much, but I figured it couldn't hurt.

Would you believe that I had my first night of sleep without a headache or achy ankles and knees? I went to bed at 11:30 p.m. and, even though I always got up in the middle of the night, I was able to get back to sleep. I finally rolled out at 9 a.m., also feeling much better.

I was feeling so good that I took a shower and went out to breakfast at my neighborhood spot. I also knew that I was going to call my nurse to ask why she did not call me back the day before. When I called to ask her about it, the nice nurse who I spoke with said she would make sure to give my nurse the message.

Within a half hour, my nurse called me back. When I told her of my displeasure, she told me she had never received my messages. I gave her the benefit of the doubt, and told her about my headache and knee and ankle pain. She told me that the headaches were caused by my anti-nausea medication, and my pains were caused by my chemo. She said she would tweak my meds on the next round, so I would not have to experience those discomforts. All this made me happy, as that was my main problem with the first round of chemo.

It was a good day as I said goodbye to the first week of my chemo treatment. The next day was April 7, and the start of week two.

CHAPTER 8

WEEK TWO

Week two started out in a good way. No problems! I was able to sleep without feeling any effects from the week before. I did know that I would be losing my hair in a week, and I was planning to have a goodbye party for it.

I decided to get a jump on it. I really did not want to go to bed and wake up the next morning with my hair on the pillow, which would freak me out. It was now Monday, April 9, and in two days, I was going to get a buzz cut. That would make the transition to baldness much easier for me.

I again remembered, when I was a little boy, telling my mother that I did not care what color my hair would be when I got older as long as I still had it. I did know that it would come back in time, plus I had reconciled with it by telling myself that should be my biggest problem.

That afternoon, I planned to walk around the park if the weather was nice. I took a walk the night before, and it felt really good. But I did tire, as I was not used to it. I was a person who worked out five days a week, and that had become a way of life for me. Since this ordeal started, I hadn't worked out for two months. I knew, when all was said and done, it would not be easy getting back up to speed.

Another thing that I noticed was that food tasted like crap, as my taste buds were also affected by the chemo. When you are a person who likes food—all kinds of food—and start having a hard time finding anything that tastes good, that became a problem. I loved pizza and was having a hard time enjoying it. Even diet soda did not taste the same. I wondered how long it would be until my taste buds returned.

On Wednesday, April 12, I was feeling good. That night, I had an appointment to have my hair buzzed. That was something that really bothered me, but I had come to the realization that it would be temporary, and my hair would eventually grow back.

I just kept looking in the mirror and putting my fingers through my hair, as a final remembrance. How I would look bald was a burning question that would be answered soon.

I checked out my stock of hats, and I had plenty of them. I had a hat from every ballpark I'd visited, from baseball to football, plus my favorites—the White Sox, Lions, Bears, and Blackhawks. I had a hat for every day of the month.

My appointment was at 6:30 p.m., so at 6 p.m. I took my final look in the mirror and headed out the door. The trip to my friend's house took me ten minutes. My friend was a stylist who did my hair in her basement salon. I figured what she had to do would not take that long.

I actually had my eyes closed when she started with the trimmers, and then some other tools. I felt my head getting colder as the hair dropped to the floor. She cut it really short so, when the rest of it fell out, it would be a smooth transition for me to become Mr. Clean.

I got my courage up to look in the mirror, and opened my eyes. I don't know why I was such a big baby with this. I figure it is because hair was something I'd always had, and seeing it gone at sixty-six was a shock to my system.

My first reaction when I saw myself was "OMG!" I was certainly glad that I did not have to look like that before. I saw a different person from the one I usually did. I don't think I ever had that little hair, even as a baby.

I felt like I might have to go around the house and cover all the mirrors once I got home. I knew that people would not see me without a hat on. I guess that I was being pretty hard on myself, but that is just the way I am.

When I got back to the house, I immediately went upstairs to my hat collection. I had to actually laugh, as most of the hats were a little big on me. I picked out my favorites, and organized them in a way where I would have a different look almost every day.

Before heading to bed, I threw out my brush, as there would be no need for one for maybe four months, and then I would just buy a new one. The next day, I would get up and go to the hospital to have my blood count tested. During chemo, your blood count is lowered and needs to be checked. You are more susceptible to infections during this time, as your immune system is compromised. This is the time that you need to be very careful. You have to make sure that you are not around any snotty people, and carry hand sanitizer with you. You cannot be too careful.

It was now Thursday, April 12, and I was headed for my blood work. In the back of my mind, I was thinking that the worst possible thing for me was any delay in my treatments. Everything hinged on my blood work that was taken today and the next week, before my second chemo treatment.

I could put my car on remote control and it would have known its way to the cancer center by now. When I got to the lab on the first floor, the order for the test was already there.

I did not have to wait very long, as I was the only person in the waiting room. The blood had to be taken out of my right hand, until the day I had no more port. The tech this time was pretty good. Sometimes you get a lab tech who used to work construction and doesn't realize that they are hurting you.

I was out of there in five minutes, and back in the car heading home. I would not find out my results until the next week. No news was good news in something like that.

The next day, April 19, I would begin my third week with my next chemo treatment. I had been feeling good after that first treatment and would probably feel the same until the next one. I was really hoping my nurse could tweak my medication like she told me she could. I was a little apprehensive about what I would feel like during round two, but I guessed time would tell.

CHAPTER 9

WEEK THREE

I didn't expect any changes this week, until my next treatment. I had been feeling pretty good, just a little tired. I usually did my routine of going out to breakfast with my paper, but now started to wear my hat and sunglasses, to go incognito. I knew that I was being foolish with this whole hair thing. But that was me, and I could not change.

I had already noticed little hair follicles on my shirt, which meant the hair I still had would soon be gone. I kidded with my friends by telling them that I'd covered all the mirrors in the house and had a hard time sleeping with a hat on. It was good that I still had my sense of humor, which had not left me throughout this ordeal.

A friend who had a different kind of cancer gave me advice and told me what to expect. Sometimes I didn't want to hear it, like when he told me that, with each dose of chemo, I would get tougher side effects. That idea bothered me, and it would be one of the questions I asked my nurse that Thursday. I hoped that my cocktail was different from his, and that my side effects would be handled in a way where I would not be that sick.

As I said earlier, I always expect the worst and hope for the best. This was my philosophy, and I was sticking to it. I could usually handle whatever life threw at me. When you don't have a choice, you just deal with it.

By that point, I didn't have the drive to go out much, except to the movie theater or to a restaurant. Thank the lord that my home was a nice size, as I found myself in many different rooms during the day. I gave all my rooms equal time, and had different shows TiVoed in different rooms. I wished I could read more, but my attention span was not great while I was going through this process.

It was Saturday, April 14, and the days were going by way too slowly for me. I wanted it to be Thursday already so I could get my second treatment and then have only two more to go. "Patience," I kept telling myself.

That night, I was supposed to go out to dinner with a friend. I did have a great support group, and was always getting calls checking up on me. People were really nice and, as they say, you know who your real friends are in tough times.

The other day, I called a friend to thank her for the chicken soup that she gave me, and told her it was really good. The next morning, when I opened the front door to go get the paper, there was a huge pot of chicken soup there.

I had another friend who came over to my house, took over the kitchen, and made me several chicken dinners. Another friend brought me frozen pizzas that were out of this world.

Then there was my daughter-in-law, who drove in from Wisconsin to sit with me during my chemo treatments, and also brought me several meals to freeze. She is an amazing cook, and everything that she made was outstanding.

I was very lucky to have such a wonderful daughter-in-law. My own daughter was pregnant and in a new job and, as much as I would have liked to have her with me, I felt it was more important that she did not have to miss work. And, with her being pregnant, I did not want her sitting with a bunch of us cancer patients. I knew that she would not be happy about it, but I made the decision for her. I wanted her pregnancy to be a happy time for her.

On Monday, April 16, I had a follow-up appointment with the breast surgeon to check out my scar and make sure everything was healing properly. The scar actually looked good, as she did an excellent job.

I almost walked out of the house without my hat. I got into the car and looked in the rearview mirror. When I saw that I was not wearing a hat, I ran back in to get it. My hat had already become part of my anatomy.

Mondays seemed to be very busy days at the surgeon's office. The waiting room was quite crowded, but again I was the only man in the room. I grabbed a cup of coffee, which tasted like shit, and waited to be called.

I waited around fifteen minutes before my name was called. I was brought into a room and told the doctor would be in shortly. Shortly turned into thirty minutes. I hated having to wait for anything. If it was a restaurant, I would have walked out.

The doctor came in and checked out her handiwork. Then we talked about hockey, as she was also a fan. I liked her, as she had great bedside manner and a great personality. Some doctors were very dry, with no sense of humor. I still had mine, and hoped that I would not lose it.

Before I left, I questioned her about my not being able to lift with my left arm, as I was afraid of lymphedema. She told me to do what I normally did and live my life, but to be careful not to lift anything heavy, like a suitcase. I still had a good right arm, so all I had to do was remember, which would be no problem.

Since I was feeling good, I took myself and my newspaper out to breakfast, per my ritual. I still missed working out but, as soon as my treatment was over, I would get back to my routine and go to my health club every day.

I just wished that these days would go by quicker than they were. Time was really dragging. I was mentally preparing myself for my second round of chemo. I knew this week would crawl until Thursday.

It was Wednesday, April 18, and tomorrow was the day that I had been waiting for—my second round. I was a little worried about it. What would my side effects be? Would they be similar? Could medication help alleviate the problems I had during the first round?

Friends told me that I was halfway through, but I felt that wouldn't be true for another three weeks. Yes, the next day the chemo treatments would be halfway through, but not the side effects.

My daughter-in-law would be arriving around noon. We would leave at 12:30 p.m., as I would have to have my blood drawn before seeing the doctor. After that, I would be taken to my cubicle and have my port accessed for my IV. The whole process would take about four and a half to five hours. Then I'd go home to relax and think about what would happen to me next.

One thing I looked forward to was my daughter-in-law bringing me several more dinners. I had never tasted anything from her that was not great and, on top of it all, the dishes were all healthy, as I was watching my carbs and sugar.

I would also bring the diary that I kept for my nurse. This way she could see how the three weeks went, and when I experienced my bad days. Everything was there, in black and white and simple to follow. I would also ask for something to help me sleep the first week afterward; it was tough to function on two hours of sleep.

So, I was ready to bring on tomorrow.

CHAPTER 10

WEEK FOUR

Tomorrow was finally here. Thursday, April 19. My daughter-in-law arrived a little early, and brought three delicious, healthy dinners for me. We wrote down our questions for my doctor and nurse, and packed the little cancer bag that I was given to keep a daily chart on how I was doing. This gave them the information on what I needed tweaked for a smoother three weeks.

Each time I went to my appointment, the first thing that had to be done was having my blood checked. I had to have the blood taken from my right hand, because I had lymph nodes out of my left arm and a port in my right arm. Some lab techs were good, and some you would think used a square needle. This time I was lucky, as the lab tech was good and it hardly hurt.

Then I was off to see my oncologist. We were taken to another room, and waited around fifteen minutes for him. It was nice to know that I had an excellent doctor. When he treated my late wife, he was able to keep her alive longer than she was expected to live.

When he walked in, he told me my blood work was very good. My white blood cell count was a high normal, which helped fight infections. The main thing was there would not be any delay in my treatment schedule. Then I asked him a very important question, which I also asked my nurse. I asked if the first treatment was an indicator of how the following three would go. So many people had told me different stories about a buildup, and how each dose would be worse. He told me that it was a very good indicator of how the others would go and that hopefully, after tweaking my meds, the side effects would be more tolerable.

After he left the room, we had to wait about ten more minutes for another nurse to bring us to my cubicle for my IV. The cubicle was very comfortable, as I sat in a recliner with my feet up.

Before my nurse came in, an aide prepared to put the IV into my port. Now, this hurt for about ten seconds, until the needle was in. Then she flushed the port and started a saline drip, followed by a syringe of anti-nausea medicine that was enough for five days.

After about half an hour of the saline drip, my nurse came in with the first part of my cocktail. The whole process took several hours, but time went fast when I had someone there to talk to.

I asked my nurse the same question I'd asked my doctor, and her answer was the same. That gave me a very good feeling. She also told me how she was tweaking my meds to try and help with my headaches, and the knee and ankle pain caused by the chemo. She called in a new prescription to the pharmacy, which I would pick up on my way home. The steroid that was also the anti-nausea medicine was what was causing my headaches. My current plan was to take two pills twice a day before chemo, two pills twice on the day of chemo, and two more the day after. The new plan was the same, except that the following day I would take only one pill, and only half a pill the day after that. I was also to take Tylenol PM, to help me sleep and ease my joint pain. I prayed that this tweaking would help me.

It was about 5 p.m., and I had finished with my second treatment. Taking the IV out was no problem. Because my blood counts were so good, I would not have to come in for a blood test before my next treatment. So off we went to the pharmacy to pick up my meds. The good news was that I only had to do this two more times.

Let me introduce you to my chemo cocktail. There were many different cocktails, but this was mine, and every oncologist I spoke with told me it had the best results. My cocktail included:

CYCLOPHOSPHAMIDE (CYTOXIN)

- Treats breast cancer and ovarian cancer, Hodgkin's disease, some leukemias, and other types of cancer.
- Slows or stops the growth of cancer cells in your body.
- Injected into the IV. This drug is usually infused over thirty minutes.
- Most common side effects — low blood counts, irritation of the bladder or kidneys, nausea, vomiting, and hair loss.
- Less common side effects — diarrhea, mouth sores, and changes in skin color.

DOCETAXEL (TAXOTERE)

- Treats breast cancer and lung cancer.
- Slows or stops the growth of cancer cells in your body.
- Infused through a tube into a vein. This drug is usually infused over a period of one hour.
- Most common side effects—low blood cell counts, hair loss, numbness or tingling in your fingers or toes, allergic-type reactions, swelling in your feet or ankles.
- Less common side effects—nausea and vomiting, diarrhea, mouth sores, aching in joints for a few days after each treatment, liver or kidney problems, skin rashes, redness and swelling followed by peeling of hands and feet.

I was lucky so far to only experience two side effects, which could hopefully be corrected. I was constantly drinking Crystal Light lemonade or water with Propel, as I didn't like regular water. It was very important to stay hydrated. I even made myself Jell-O and drank chicken broth.

If it went like the last session, I would be okay the next day and start feeling the side effects on Sunday. Time would tell.

Meanwhile, my hair was almost all out, and I was still having a hard time adjusting to the new look. A few people close to me had seen me without my hat, and said I did not look bad. Either they were being nice—who would tell someone that they looked like shit?—or they were being honest. Everyone said that I was too hard on myself, which I probably was. I did ask how fast the hair would come back. I was told that, after a few weeks when chemo was over, the hair would come back at about a quarter inch per month. If it would help it grow faster, I would rub some fertilizer on my hair and water it. Oh well, it is what it is.

It was now Saturday, April 21, the day before the side effects were to hit. I was anxious to see if the slight change in my meds would help. I had no problems since my Thursday treatment. I did lose more hair, and felt like I looked like a hard-boiled egg with eyes. I was constantly drinking fluids to stay hydrated.

Saturday was a rather good day. It was my son's birthday. I watched a perfectly pitched game by my White Sox, and finished the day by watching my Blackhawks win an overtime playoff game.

I wanted to make sure that I'd get a good night's sleep because I was not sure if I would be able to sleep for the next three days. I planned to stay up a little longer, to make sure I'd get good and tired. I was waiting to see what tomorrow would be like. At least this round, I knew what to expect. My fingers were crossed.

Sunday was day four after my chemo treatment. After the last treatment, it took until the third day for it to hit me, so it was like waiting for the other shoe to drop. I went to bed Saturday night thinking I would feel something the next day. I actually had a rather good sleep and rolled out of bed at 10 a.m., feeling pretty good. Not even as tired as I was the day before. I could not figure this out. Maybe the tweaking of my meds had something to do with it.

So I got my behind out of bed and, since I was feeling good, I wanted to take advantage of it and took myself out for breakfast with my newspaper. In the back of my mind, I thought that something was not right, as I felt too good. I figured that, if I felt good for a few more days, then I might be out of the woods on this round.

I even started to plan a party called a "Celebration Of Life," which would be my way of thanking everyone for their support and caring while I went through this ordeal. I loved parties, and had them for any good reason I could find. In this case, a party like this would definitely beat a funeral.

I rolled out of bed the next morning at 9:30 a.m., and still felt pretty good. Sunday night, I had a very minor pain in my legs caused by the chemo, but it was so minor that it was really not worth mentioning. This was the fifth day after the treatment, and I was still waiting for something to happen. Like I said previously, I was in unchartered water and didn't really know what to expect.

It was a beautiful day, so I was going to have lunch with a friend and get out of the house, and maybe go to an afternoon matinee. When I was feeling good, I wanted to do something, and just had a hard time sitting around. I really wanted to go back to the health club but, with my resistance still low, I did not want to take a chance with all the germs at the club. Better safe than sorry, as far as that went.

My best rest was usually from 6 a.m. until I rolled out of bed. Wednesday, I rolled out at 10:12 a.m. I had only minor discomfort in my legs, which did not stop me from sleeping. I got up and felt good enough to do my breakfast routine.

While sitting in my booth reading the paper, I suddenly felt very tired. This was the fatigue the doctors talked about.

♦ *Richard W. Wiener*

I sat there until I felt strong enough to get up, pay my check, and leave. I'd intended to do some grocery shopping but, for the second day in a row, made the decision to just go home. It was not that I didn't have food in the house, but shopping gave me something to do.

So I drove back home and took my place on the couch. It was Wednesday, April 25, and I was finishing my fourth week of chemo. I wanted to bring on tomorrow, so I could begin week five.

PHOTO ALBUM

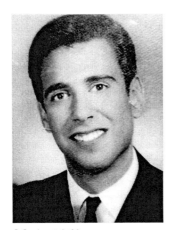

Me in 1968.

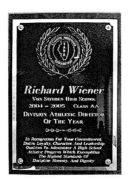

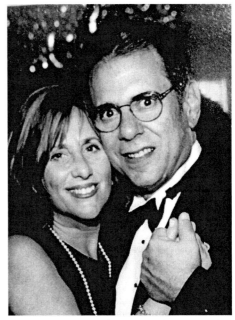

With my late wife Lynn who passed away in 2007 from breast cancer

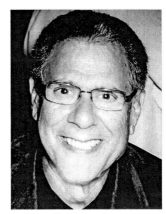

I actually have hair.

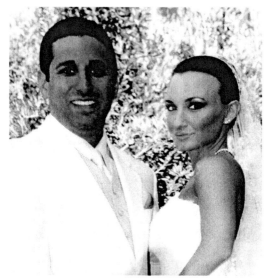

My son Chad and Katy at their wedding.

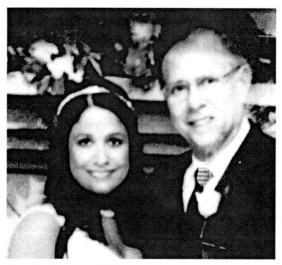

On Amber's wedding day.

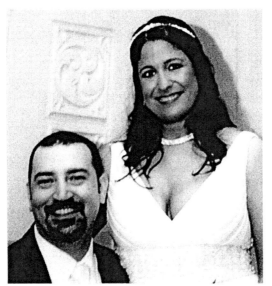

My daughter Amber and her husband Frank on their wedding day

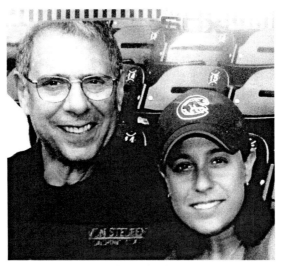

Amber and myself at a ball game

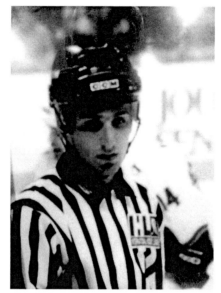

Chad during his hockey official days.

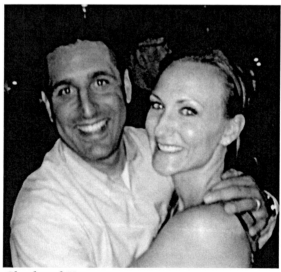

Chad and Katy.

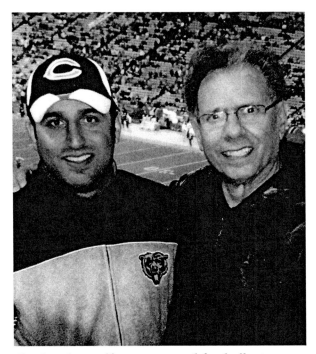

Chad and myself at our annual football trip.

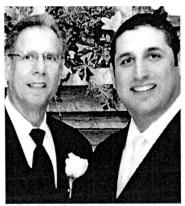

Chad and me.

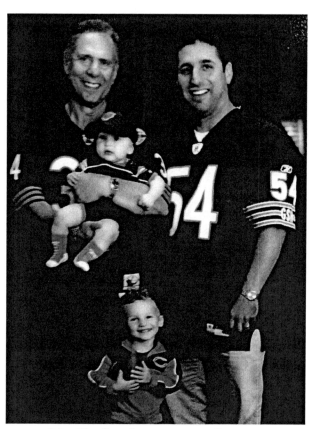

Me, Chad and my two grandsons.

CHAPTER 11

WEEK FIVE

Fatigue! Now I knew what it really felt like. For the last two days, I felt so exhausted that it was hard to even walk up the stairs to the bedroom. This was a major side effect of chemo and one that everyone has to deal with. I kept asking myself, how do people work when they are totally fatigued? I was fortunate that I had no job, and my main objective was just to get well.

This was the beginning of week five. I wished it would go faster, as I got really bored with nothing to do or nowhere to go. But the main thing was that I was feeling a little better today than I had the last two days. This was the routine. I would start to get better and, when I felt really good, it would be time for the next treatment.

I was looking forward to that night, as I had a meeting that I must attend. Also, the next night I was having dinner with some friends who had not seen me since this all started. Then, over the weekend, my son and daughter-in-law would be coming in from Milwaukee to go out to dinner. I always loved to have things to look forward to.

It was Thursday, April 26, seven days since my last chemo, and I was starting to feel much better. I was figuring out this pattern, and now I thought I knew what to expect.

I knew that when all this was over, I would have to get myself back on a normal schedule again. I wanted to be able to get out of bed at 9 a.m. and go to the health club at 10 a.m. No more getting out of bed at 10 or 10:30.

Another thing that I was looking forward to was food tasting like food again. Right now, everything tasted like shit. Even coffee and diet soda. My favorite food was pizza, and I knew there was a problem when even that tasted like shit. The only thing that tasted the way it should was water.

It was 2 p.m. and my meeting was at 6 p.m., so I just rested to conserve my energy. Maybe I'd take a nap, which I rarely did.

I made it through my meeting, but could not wait to get back home. A tiredness just crept up on me without any warning. It was around 9:30 p.m. when I opened my door to the house. I got undressed and sat on my couch with my remote control. A most familiar sight. Around 11:30 p.m., I headed upstairs to watch the TV in my room. I usually watched TV until I got tired enough to go to sleep.

I wished that I could go to sleep. I was up every two hours no matter what. The clock seemed to never move. A pattern was developing where I'd finally get my best sleep from around 5 a.m. until I finally got out of bed anywhere from 10-10:30 a.m. It didn't bother me, as I had nowhere to go, and each day was the same.

The next day, I met a friend for lunch and lasted about an hour before I hit the wall. I expected to start to feeling better any day now. That was, if the pattern was the same. I also hoped to finally meet some friends for dinner, something that I had not yet done. We were going to my favorite chicken place, which I normally liked. I knew everything would still taste like shit, but it would be good to get out.

So I would again try to conserve my energy by trying to take a nap. Maybe, just maybe, I could get about an hour or two of shuteye. Again, my fingers were crossed.

Dinner was good, even though I could not really taste the chicken. It was good to get out of the house. I lasted about two hours and then I started to get tired so, knowing my body, I said it was time to go.

So once back at the house, I put myself on the famous couch and watched my favorite programs. Around 11 p.m., I decided to head upstairs to watch more TV and maybe fall asleep. When that happened, I would know that I was over the hump of round two. Around 1 a.m., I decided to take two Tylenol PM to help me sleep.

I must have been up every hour until around 6 a.m. Then I fell asleep, and opened my eyes around 8 a.m. I couldn't get out of bed so, having nothing to do, I stayed there until 11 a.m. At that time, I rolled out of bed and got myself ready for another wonderful day.

I was meeting a friend and his wife at a restaurant in my neighborhood at 2 p.m., and then I would head to the grocery store and do some food shopping. I was tired before I left the house, but the cool breeze woke me up and actually felt good.

Lunch was nice, and the conversation was good. I ordered a French onion soup, another food I loved that now tasted like dirt. Nothing tasted good to me. I stopped drinking coffee, as that was the worst. Even diet soda tasted tinny.

After lunch, I went to the grocery store and bought things that I would need for the week. I passed up a lot of things I normally bought, because I knew what they would taste like.

So now I was back at home and back in my position. I would be in that same position for the night, as even a movie didn't thrill me enough to get me out of the house.

Tomorrow, my son and daughter-in-law would be coming from Milwaukee to have dinner with me. I was looking forward to that, as I loved spending time with them.

It was Saturday, April 28, nine days into round two. Any day now, I should begin to feel better. Maybe it would be tomorrow.

This could be the day. I only got up once Saturday night, slept until 9:30 a.m. Sunday, and got up feeling refreshed. I had been waiting for this day, and it took until the tenth day for my body to start feeling good.

I felt so good that I took myself hat shopping. Most of my hats were too big on me. I wanted to check out the styles, as I wanted one for dress and one for everyday. I found what I was looking for at Target. I made my big purchase and headed home to relax and take a shower. I still found it strange having the water beat down on my hairless head, but it actually felt pretty good. And it was easy to dry off with the swipe of a towel.

The timing couldn't have been better, as that night my kids were coming from Wisconsin to have dinner with me at one of our favorite places, Wildfire. I made reservations for 4:30 p.m., which would give us more than ample time to sit and relax and, with a sitter for my two grandsons, that would allow my son to get back home in a timely manner.

Usually, I would start thinking about what I wanted for dinner but now, with food tasting as it did to me, it would make no difference what I ordered. Whether it was a dirt salad, a dirt steak, or a dirt piece of fish, everything would taste the same. Just like dirt. I stopped complaining as nothing would change, and I was sure people were getting tired of it. So from then on, I would say nothing. Bring on my skirt steak.

Dinner was really nice. Good conversation with good company. Everyone loved their dinner and I would have also, but the taste was not there. I ordered my usual skirt steak, but need I say more?

We sat and talked for more than two hours, and I was starting to get a little tired. I guessed people could tell by my eyes when I started getting tired. My eyes began to get glossy and feel heavy. I also became rather quiet, and all the signals were there that my evening was coming to an end. So my son went back to Wisconsin, and I went back to my couch.

The next two days were the same, as I felt pretty good and my sleeping went back to normal. I would get up at 9 a.m. and start my day, instead of at 11 a.m. I could not wait until I got back to my regular schedule of getting up and heading to the health club, then to breakfast. I sure hoped it wasn't going to be hard getting back into my normal routine.

It was Tuesday, May 1, and I was happy to get April behind me. I could see the light at the end of the tunnel. Two treatments in May and, by the end of June, I would hopefully start to feel like myself.

I had nothing planned for this week. I could go to a movie or out to dinner. Actually, I would probably go out the next afternoon, as I had my cleaning crew coming in to clean the house. I hated being home when they were there, as I felt that I was in the way. Usually three women comprised the crew, and each one took a floor, which had me scrambling. So it was easier for me to just get out and go somewhere for a few hours. So a matinee it would be.

CHAPTER 12

WEEK SIX

It was Friday, May 4, and, for the first time since the last treatment, I was feeling good. I had gone through a period of being tired all the time. My sleeping was screwed up, as I would fall asleep at 3 or 4 a.m., and could not get out of bed until 10 or 11 a.m. As soon as I would get out of bed, I knew how I would feel for the day.

Today I felt good and, hopefully, I would feel the same way until next Thursday's treatment. A week of feeling good was a blessing during this time. One thing that hadn't changed was that food still tasted like shit.

Last night I had a pizza, and was hoping that my sense of taste had returned. Well, needless to say, it did not. So I had one piece and froze the rest, for when I could get the real taste of it.

I should have been losing weight, but not being able to work out — coupled with sitting on the couch or lying down all the time — worked against me losing any weight. I ate so I didn't lose any strength.

The other night, a friend came over and we went for a rather long walk. It felt good to get out and just walk. We must have walked for two miles, which was the longest that I had walked since before everything started in February. At the end of the walk, my legs were feeling like Jell-O, but I made it. The next day, I had an especially hard time getting out of bed. It was still worth it, and I looked forward to doing it again.

So now I was deciding what I should do for the day, since I was feeling good. Maybe a movie or a walk in the mall. I could always go hat shopping, as I was looking at different hats and not just baseball hats. Most of my hats were a tad too big. I wished that I was not as hard on myself as I was. If I did not look decent, I felt I could not leave the house.

I had to find a hat to wear for a June 23 wedding that I responded to. Was there such a thing as a dress hat? I needed one that would go with a dark suit. My favorite Blackhawks hat would not go with my outfit. Now I was on a mission.

Despite my plans, I never made it out of the house Friday because of the weather. It turned cool and rainy, so

I decided that my mission would wait until the next nice day. The important thing was that I was feeling good. Good enough where I met some friends for dinner Friday night.

We went to a nice restaurant, but it was the same result for me when it came to taste. It could be fish, steak, chicken, or even pizza, it all tasted like you-know-what. So I decided on skirt steak.

After dinner, I headed home to watch some TV and then try to go to sleep. I turned off the TV at 1:30 a.m. and tried to fall asleep. It might have been about 2:30 a.m. when I fell asleep. When I opened my eyes, it was four hours later, but way too early for me to get up. I stayed in bed until 9:45 a.m. and decided to get up and get ready to go out to breakfast.

It was Saturday May 5, and I was feeling good. Five more days until my next treatment, which would be the halfway point. I was hoping that the week would go by fast.

Sunday, May 6 was a rainy day. I had nothing planned for the day, and would do what I did best—sit on the couch and watch the ballgame. The only time I would go out of the house would be to get the Sunday papers from the front lawn. The biggest decision that I would make would be what I should eat for brunch and dinner. I did not go to my usual breakfast place on Sunday, as it was too crowded and I could not wait for a table.

I was feeling good and counting the days until Thursday, when I would be at the halfway point of my treatment. I wished I could just wiggle my nose and get rid of May and June, then be on my way to being my old self.

Monday morning, I was meeting a friend for a late breakfast. I looked forward to having something to do. There were just way too many down days for me.

It was almost midnight and I would probably take two Tylenol PM to help me sleep. I planned to roll out of bed at 10 a.m. and leave the house at 10:30 a.m. Maybe I would walk around the mall in the afternoon. It looked like another wonderful day in paradise.

I had another tough night sleeping. I did not think I strung more than two hours together. Even when I was able to sleep, it was not very good. I kept wishing these weeks away.

So I rolled out of bed at 9:30 a.m. I was meeting my friend at 11 a.m., so I go out front to grab my paper, and made a cup of coffee in my Keurig. The coffee tasted funny, like everything else I put in my mouth.

I left at 10:30 a.m. and headed for the restaurant. It was nice seeing my friend, who told me that I looked good without hair. I had a hard time excepting that, as I was still not used to my new look. Maybe I would spray paint my head.

I even ordered a few new hats online, which would arrive in a few days. Hopefully I could find one that I really liked. I still needed a dress hat for the wedding in June.

After breakfast, I had an errand to run and then headed home. I actually fell asleep on the couch for an hour, which felt good. Then I had to make a major decision. What should I have for dinner? I decided to go out, as I looked for any excuse to leave the house when I felt good.

After dinner, I went home and got into my favorite position to watch a ballgame and other programs that I'd recorded. I was getting close to Thursday, the halfway point. Two more days to go. Maybe I could sleep tonight.

I got out of bed Wednesday at 10:15 a.m., and felt really good. So good that I went out to breakfast and ran some errands. At night, I was going to see a play and have dinner. I found it amazing how one day I felt like shit, and the next day I felt normal.

The afternoon passed really quickly. I met a friend for dinner, and then we went to the play. It was quite enjoyable. Dinner was okay, as I still could not taste the real flavor.

I got home at 10:30 p.m. and put on one of my favorite programs that I'd TiVoed—"American Idol," which I never missed. It was over around midnight, as I fast forwarded through the commercials. The funny thing was that I was not tired.

At 3:30 a.m., I was wide awake. This was the part that I did not like. My sleeping was still all messed up. Pills did not even help. It was the same thing before the last chemo session. I did not know why I was not nervous, but I was more anxious to get in and get out. I was also excited about what my daughter-in-law was bringing me for my dinners.

    I was going to try to get to sleep. I even set my alarm for 9:30 a.m., but knew that I would be up way before my cell alarm went off. I wanted to get up, shower, have my coffee, read the paper, and relax before my daughter-in-law arrived at noon. I had my blood test at 12:30 p.m. and, before I sat down for chemo, I would see the doctor at 1 p.m.

    Yep, tomorrow I would be at the halfway mark. Yeah!

CHAPTER 13

WEEK SEVEN

I arrived for my blood test at 12:30 p.m. They had to take blood from my right hand, and that stung a little. When they tell you it will feel like a bee sting, picture a fifty-pound bee taking a bite out of you.

Then I was brought into a room to see the doctor. He already had my blood report, which came out very good. He told me that I was doing great and looked great. We talked about the BRCA test, which I would take after my treatment was over. This test would tell me if I was a genetic risk for cancer. I asked him if I was an automatic positive since I had cancer and, surprisingly, he said no. I had an 80 percent chance of being negative and a 20 percent chance of being positive. I was not great with these percentages as, remember, that only 1 percent of breast cancers happen to men, and I was one of them. If I tested positive, then my children would have to be tested. If I was negative, then no one had to be tested.

I asked the doctor when I could have my port taken out, and he told me that it would come out about five weeks after treatment ended. I would then be put on the drug tamoxifen for five years. I was also to see the doctor every three months to get checked.

The four hours of chemo passed quickly, as my daughter-in law went over the menu for my "Celebration of Life" party, which she was catering. She was such a fabulous cook, she could make dog food taste like a filet. We went over a theme for the party, as she was also very creative.

Before I knew it, the buzzer started ringing, telling my nurse that I was finished and could leave. That night I would take it easy, and attempt to go to the health club the next day. My nurse told me to go and work out, as that was the best way to fight fatigue. So that night I would take two Tylenol PM and try to get some much-needed sleep. Then I would get up at 9 a.m., be at the club at 10 a.m., and then go to my breakfast place. I really hoped it would help with the fatigue. My fingers were crossed.

I woke up Friday morning after a decent night's sleep. I was feeling really good, as I knew I would for the next few days. So I took advantage of it by getting up and going to the health club. I must say that it felt great to somewhat get back to my regular routine.

The first time back at the club since the beginning of February, I did not want to push myself too hard. I walked for thirty minutes and totaled a mile and a half. I walked at a slower clip than I normally did, and would work back up to my normal pace.

Then I headed for my breakfast place, where I read my paper and enjoyed the morning. I got back home around noon and started doing work on my computer. I had to take advantage of the times when I was feeling good. My spirits were good and my belief that you always had to have something to look forward to kept me going. I was really excited about my "Celebration of Life" party in November.

That night I was going out to dinner with the guys. It was Friday, May 11, and it was a good day.

I had a pretty good night's sleep, but not as good as the other night. I still woke up feeling okay, which I expected. I knew from what I felt the last time that the fatigue wouldn't really hit me until the third or fourth day. But this time, I had a game plan, which was to fight that fatigue by continuing to exercise.

Saturday morning I went to the club again, and walked 1.6 miles in thirty-five minutes. I hoped to slowly build that back up to where I was before this ordeal started. Once back home, I was in my relaxed mode. One thing I noticed was that I was very thirsty. For breakfast, I did not have coffee, which still tasted like mud, and instead had a pitcher of water. I was told that, for the first five days after chemo, I should consume sixty-four ounces of water a day. So water was by me all day long.

Depending on how I felt that night, I might go to dinner with a friend or go to a movie. I might even stay in to watch the ballgame. The next day was Mother's Day and, if I felt okay, I would go to the cemetery to visit my mother's grave and tell her about my ordeal. It was Saturday, May 12, and I had started my countdown to my last treatment on May 31.

―――――――

Sunday was Mother's Day, and I was still feeling pretty good. This was day three after chemo, and my fatigue usually began on the fourth or fifth day.

I was going to do what I usually did on this day, and that was make my cemetery rounds. I had to drive about forty minutes to get to the cemetery that my immediate family was in, and then travel back to visit my late wife. Then I would go to breakfast with paper in hand. I hoped that I wouldn't have to wait long, as the restaurant got quite busy on Sunday, plus it was Mother's Day.

After breakfast, I would go home and assume my position on the couch to watch more sporting events. I slept reasonably well last night considering I took a few pills, but still got up to pee like a racehorse because of all the fluids I drank during the day.

The next day was Monday May 14, and the fourth day after chemo, so I was still going to get up and go to the club. My fingers were crossed.

What a difference a day made. Rough night Sunday night. I was quite tired, but could not fall asleep. I took two Tylenol PM and had no results so, at 4 a.m., I took one of the pills given to me by my nurse. That seemed to work, as I did fall asleep and could not get out of bed until 10:45 a.m.

I did not have the energy to go to the health club, probably because I took a long walk the night before. I did have a dull ache in my knees and right ankle, but it was very tolerable. At least there were no headaches. So today I was staying in and lying low, and expected to be like that for a few days. The key was a decent night's sleep. If I could get that, then I would try the health club tomorrow. I was also really thirsty, so I was still constantly drinking and peeing like a racehorse.

But my thoughts were all positive, as I was in the second half of my treatment and counting the days until May 31. Hopefully, that would be the last time I would have to sit in the chemo chair.

I was hoping that Monday night would be different from Sunday night. My fingers were crossed again.

Last night was not very good, but pretty bad. Sleeping pills did not work, and I had some discomfort in my knees and legs. I started out in my bed and ended up on the basement couch. At 8 a.m., I got off the couch and went back to my bed to watch TV. I stayed there until 10 a.m., and then got up. Since I seemed to be feeling a little better, I went to do some banking and then out to breakfast.

I should have been used to this by then. I wanted to go for a walk, as it was a beautiful day, but my knees might not allow that. Maybe a little later when I saw how I felt. It seemed to worsen as the day went on. But I knew that in a matter of a few days, this would pass and I'd only have one more treatment to endure this feeling.

The most disturbing part to me was sleeping. If I could only get decent rest at night, then maybe my days would be better. It was Tuesday, May 15, and so far it was a little better than yesterday.

I slept a little better last night after I took two pills. I felt good enough to go out to lunch, see a movie, and do some grocery shopping. I had to force myself out of the house, as my cleaning girls were there today.

I had been experiencing some discomfort in my knees and ankles due to the chemo. I knew it would be gone in a day. At least I had no headaches, which I'd had after round one.

One thing that really annoyed me was that I had a horrible taste in my mouth. No matter what I drank, I could not get rid of it. It made me not want to eat. I tried different drinks, with no success. This was a new problem that I hadn't had before. If I thought food tasted bad before, I could only imagine what it would taste like now. I decided I just might drink my dinner that night.

Tonight I would just stay in and do my usual thing—nothing. I would take two pills again before I tried to go to sleep and hope that tonight would be better than last night. Tomorrow, I would start on another week.

CHAPTER 14

WEEK EIGHT

Another bad night last night, as I could not get this horrible taste out of my mouth. I must say that this round was kicking my ass, and I could only imagine what round four would be like.

I did not get out of bed until 11 a.m., and jumped into the shower, hoping that the water over my head would make me feel good. I also threw a load of laundry into the machine and did my daily chores. I was moving around slowly, not knowing what today would bring. I had nothing really planned, except driving my son to the airport in the late afternoon.

I seemed to get through the days, but those nights were what bothered me. All I wanted was to get a good night's sleep without getting up six times. No one should ever take feeling great for granted! I was praying that today would be better than yesterday, and I would know soon.

I seemed to be getting a little better. That horrendous taste was gone from my mouth. I actually had a taste for some hot and sour soup, which I ordered. It was good and spicy, and hit the spot.

The best thing was that I was feeling tired, and turned off the TV and lights at 11 p.m. For me, that was really early, but I did manage to get a good night's sleep. Of course, I did not sleep all the way through. I got up a few times, but I did manage to go back to sleep.

I opened my eyes at 9 a.m. and stayed in bed until 9:30 a.m., and then got up. I seemed to feel better than the day before, which seemed to fit the pattern. I felt good enough to have a battery replaced in my watch and go out to breakfast.

While eating breakfast, I started to get tired. Amazing how fast I got drained of energy. I finished my breakfast and sat in my booth, waiting to gather my strength to get up and go home.

After about ten minutes, I picked myself up, paid my check, and headed to my car for the short ride home. The only thing I felt was tired. If I could get some strength back in the afternoon, I might join some friends for Friday night dinner.

It was May 18, and I was thirteen days away from round four. It could not come soon enough. It is funny; when you want time to go slow, it never does and, when you want it to speed up, it goes at a snail's pace.

It seemed that my appetite was not what it used to be. I sat on my couch and watched TV the rest of the day and evening. I turned in around 11 p.m. and tried to fall asleep. It took so damn long to fall asleep and finally, around 4 a.m., I fell asleep and had my best rest.

It was 10:15 a.m. when I got up to start my day. As with most days, my morning energy was greater than in the afternoon. I decided to do a few errands, go out to lunch, and then see a movie. By 3:30 p.m., my energy was leaving my body. I came home after the movie and put myself in my most famous position.

Being tired or fatigued was the only side effect left from this round. I did believe the worst was over. At least, I prayed that the worst was over. I would watch TV and warm up some dinner later. I actually had to get up around 8:30 a.m. the next morning, as I had to pick my kids up at the airport from their weekend in Boston.

On the way home, we would stop and pick up a few cases of water. I could not lift them, so that way my son could carry them. Then we would stop for breakfast before we came to my house and they could start their drive back to Milwaukee.

It was Sunday, May 20. The alarm on my cell phone went off at 8:30 a.m. I jumped out of bed, as I was not used to an alarm getting me up. I was feeling okay, but I usually did in the morning. I got dressed and waited for the message that the plane had landed.

I was reading the paper when the message came through at 9 a.m. that the plane had arrived. I then left for the airport and picked up my kids. It was nice hearing about all the details of their weekend in Boston. I had been there a few years ago, and remembered some of the places they went.

On the way home, we stopped at the grocery store so I could get three cases of water. Then we came back home. My son unloaded the water and, before I knew it, they were on their way back home.

I was feeling pretty good and did some laundry before I started to run out of energy. I then hit the couch and watched the ballgame. I wanted to rest, as I had four friends coming over that night for dinner and to watch a movie in my theater.

I figured that we would order Chinese food instead of pizza. I had a craving for hot and sour soup, as I could taste the spice in it. It would feel good to have some people over, as I was starting to get really bored. I was ten days out from the last treatment, and finally starting to feel somewhat normal. Yeah me!

It was great having company over, as I needed the social interaction. They came over at 5:30 p.m. and stayed until 11 p.m. I then headed upstairs to watch some TV and, around midnight, I shut it off and closed my eyes.

―――――

What a good night's sleep I had. The best in a long time. I got up once around 2 a.m. and, the next thing I knew, it was 10:30 a.m. When my eyes opened, I knew that I had more energy and did not have to wait until my legs hit the ground.

While still in bed, I planned my day. I would go to the bank, then the health club, and then breakfast. A normal beginning to a day. I was hoping that I would feel the same for the next ten days until May 31.

I walked a mile and a half on the treadmill in thirty minutes. At the end, I was feeling a little tired, but I was not surprised. Breakfast even tasted good. I had an egg wrap that actually tasted like an egg wrap. I stayed around for an hour, finishing my paper, and started to feel like I was losing energy. So home I went. If I rested and felt energized later, I would see what was playing at the theater five minutes away. If it was something I wanted to see, then I would go tonight or maybe tomorrow. Just had to see how I felt.

―――――

I stayed in that day after my exhausting morning and had another decent night's rest. Today was Tuesday, May 22, and I was going to try something different. I was thinking that I did way too much, as I hadn't exercised regularly in months and should not have gone the speed or time that I did. I should have worked gradually up to where I wanted to be.

Since I had my morning energy, I decided I would only walk for twenty minutes at a lesser speed, and see how that went. I was just trying to regulate myself and get in some exercise. It was a way of life for me before all this started.

I did my twenty minutes, called it a day, and went to lunch. While at lunch, my energy left me again. I guessed my body was not ready for this. I was trying to do as I was told and push myself, but the drained feeling was just not worth it.

I scrubbed the rest of my plans for going to the grocery store and maybe a movie. Instead, I traded those plans for a place on my beloved couch. I was getting used to this and could not wait until my last treatment. After that, I would know that when I felt good, it would last, as there would be no fifth treatment. Just healing my body and then working back to where I was when this all started. These days seemed to be getting longer for me, but I was only nine days away from my last treatment.

I was so tired of being tired. Today I stayed in bed until 10:30 a.m. and wanted to conserve my energy, as I had an awards ceremony that I wanted to attend at night. So the only thing I would do until I left in the afternoon would be to go out to lunch and come home.

It really made no difference, as I was still tired and could not shake the feeling of not being myself. But I would force myself to get dressed, meet everyone for dinner, and then go to the high school. This would be the first time in sixteen years that I would not be a presenter at the ceremony. At least I would be there to observe.

Tomorrow would be fourteen days since the last treatment, and I wondered how long it would be before I started to feel better. After all, my next treatment was next Thursday and, after the way this one had gone, I was expecting the worst. The next month would be really long.

One thing I had noticed was that, when I felt this way, my eyes became glassy. When that cleared up, I knew that it would be a sign of getting better.

So I mustered up some strength and got dressed for the ceremony. I hadn't even left yet, but was already looking forward to getting home.

CHAPTER 15

WEEK NINE

I made it through last night with ease. I had enough gas in my tank to go out to dinner and make the entire ceremony, which lasted until 9:30 p.m. It was good to get home and just sit on the couch and watch what I'd TiVoed.

I had a good night's rest and seemed to feel energized today, but I had felt that way before and ran out of steam really quick. Each day was a new day, and I always hoped for the best.

So today began week nine, with a few more to go. One more treatment next week, followed by what I anticipated would be three really tough weeks. Then a final visit to the doctor, until I had to come back in to get checked.

I began my day with breakfast and then, who knew what. It was not like I scheduled a ton of things to do. How I felt after I ate would determine my afternoon.

I did feel much better. I made a discovery about the way I felt. Every day that I was tired and felt fatigued, I noticed that my eyes were very watery. Today they were not, and I felt more normal. Watery eyes were a true sign for me that I had to take it easy and rest.

I felt good enough to go out to dinner with a friend and sit outside, as it was a beautiful night. I came home after, watched some TV, and went to sleep around 12:30 a.m.

I rolled out of bed at 10 a.m., and my eyes were still clear. They would probably stay that way until next Thursday. The next time they cleared up, I would know that I was on my way to healing from the chemo.

Today I would do something that I had not done in a while, but was way overdue—get a pedicure. I always felt good after I had one, so why not take advantage of the way I was feeling and just go do it? Then it would be out to lunch and then home, as I planned on meeting some friends for dinner tonight.

It was Friday May 25, and I was feeling good. I was looking forward to when I could say that every day. The light was at the end of the tunnel, but I thought I could see it.

It was always good to be out in a social setting after being home and not feeling well for weeks. I had a few more days and planned to take advantage of them. Dinner was good, even though the food still tasted like crap. Just being out was the main thing. I was still not comfortable having no hair. It would be a huge day when I could go out without wearing a hat.

I got home around 10 p.m. and did not retire until around midnight, as usual. Tomorrow was Saturday, and another day closer to the finish line.

I just couldn't get out of bed Saturday morning, as it was raining and thundering. Plus, I had nothing to do. I was feeling good, which was the most important thing. When I felt good, I'd get really bored, especially when I had no plans scheduled.

When it stopped raining, I would go out front and get my paper, then make the decision for the day. Where should I go to lunch? That was the extent of my decision making for one day.

Weekends were harder than weekdays, as I was so used to doing something on the weekends. I wished I could look in the mirror and watch my hair grow back but, as everyone told me, it would eventually.

It looked like it had stopped raining, so out I went to get my paper and then start my wonderful Saturday.

Saturday turned out to be a good day. I spent the day watching the ballgame, and then met a friend for dinner and a movie. I did not get home until 11 p.m.

I would have liked to report that I slept like a baby, but that was not the case. I tossed and turned until 4 a.m., then fell asleep and rolled out of bed at 10:45 a.m. on Sunday.

It was Sunday, May 27, and I was feeling good. I did have plans at night, as a friend would be coming over for dinner and a walk or a movie. During the day, I would rest and conserve my energy. I was not going out to breakfast and would just have something at home. The Sunday paper would keep me occupied for a while, and then the ballgame would start. This had the makings of a decent day, and I did not get enough of those.

It was a good day yesterday. I still had the tired feeling, but I was able to go out to dinner and come back home to watch a movie with a friend.

The hard part, again, was getting to sleep. I stayed up late to get super tired, but it took me a few hours to go to sleep. At my appointment on Thursday, I needed to ask for a sleeping pill. I didn't like taking them, but felt that I had no choice.

I stayed in bed this morning as long as I could. After all, I had nowhere to go. I had no plans today, but tonight a friend would be coming over and we would go to a movie.

The weather was very hot out, so it would be the air conditioning for me, as the hot weather zapped any energy that I had. Plus, when I had something planned, I tried to conserve my energy. I was still waiting for the day when I felt like I used to feel before everything started. Everyone told me that it would happen, but I couldn't wait. The year was almost half over, and what a half year it had been for me. At least I was here to tell about it.

It was another horrible night last night. I really needed a sleeping pill. I went from the bedroom to the basement, and back to the bedroom. It is a terrible feeling when you are so tired but cannot fall asleep. With my other two treatments, I would start to feel good a few days before the next treatment. But this time, I had not felt good at all, and the next treatment was in two days. I could only imagine what I was going to be like in the fourth round. I anticipated the worst, and hoped for the best.

The only thing I had planned for the whole month was meeting up with my kids at the racetrack June 13, for Father's Day. That would be two weeks after my final treatment. My fingers were crossed that I could make it.

Nothing was going on today for me. Tonight I was meeting friends for dinner. The thing I dreaded was attempting to go to sleep. I was starting to think I would never feel normal again. It was Tuesday, May 29, and the days were going slower and slower.

I actually slept last night. What a relief. Today I had to leave the house, as my cleaning girls were coming in around noon. I figured they'd be gone by 3 p.m., and decided to take myself out to the mall and maybe a movie. Tonight I was having dinner with a friend, so today would hopefully go fast. I also had to start my pills, as tomorrow was my final round of chemo.

I did feel that I had a little more energy today. I had seen it get drained in a very short period of time before, but today I would push myself, as I expected that round four would be the worst one and would keep me in the house most of the time. I really hoped that I was wrong.

It was now 2:45 p.m., and the cleaning crew was gone. The movie was good, and I still felt okay. I now had time to relax before I got picked up at 6:45 p.m. for dinner. I was looking forward to tomorrow, as that would be the last time I would have to use my port. I was also anxious to hear about my followups and any scans that I might have to take in the future. Also, I wanted to know when I would start taking tamoxifen. And I had to make sure to ask my nurse about a sleeping pill, as I really need one for the next round.

CHAPTER 16

WEEK TEN

Today was the day, but last night was just like the night before my previous treatments. Zero sleep. I turned off my light and TV at 2 a.m., and did not get even a minute of sleep. So now it was 7 a.m., and I just decided to get out of bed. It would be a long morning for me. My daughter-in-law would not be there until noon, so I did what I did the last time—go out to breakfast, then come home, sit on the couch, and watch morning TV.

It was a rainy spring day, and my daughter-in-law got stuck in traffic, so she met me at the doctor's office. I did my usual routine of having blood drawn from my right hand, which took three minutes. Each time I got a new lab person, and hoped they were good. Some had such light touches, and some were like construction workers. Today's was just fine.

Next step was up one floor to the oncology department. There I filled out my questionnaire asking me if I had any side effects, as each round was different. When they saw one, they could try to adjust the meds to help. My main concern was sleep deprivation.

Now I was taken into a room to wait for my doctor. I always took the first appointment, so I did not have to wait long. At 1:10 p.m., he came in. My first question to him was when I would start feeling good, as I was so tired of being tired. I was told that I should feel almost myself in six weeks, and that was when he would like to see me for a follow-up appointment. He told me that I got zapped with a heavy-duty drug, and he did it in four weeks because I could handle it. Some cases were marathons and some were sprints. Mine was a sprint, which I preferred.

He told me that I would not need radiation and that, by the beginning of September, I would have a short, crew-cut look on my head. Also, when I saw him again, I would make an appointment to have my port removed from my arm. I would then see him once every three months to get checked and go on tamoxifen for five years. This was all fine with me, as I would be checked all the time, where many people were walking around unchecked.

Once I felt better, I would tackle the colonoscopy that was overdue because of the current problem. But, rest assured, there would not be a book on that one.

When I saw the nurse who gave me the chemo IV, she told me that this could be the toughest round. I figured that, as the third round was not good for three weeks. The first day I felt good was the day I got zapped again. But this time, I was getting a sleeping pill, and I prayed that it would work. I was told to be patient and not to get depressed, as this was the part when people did get depressed, because they were not feeling better fast enough. I would not get depressed, as I saw the light at the end of the tunnel, and it was getting larger.

So on my way home, I stopped to pick up my pills, then headed home to order out dinner. Today was Thursday, and I figured by Sunday my tiredness would hit me and continue for the next three weeks or so. As always, I expected the worst and hoped for the best.

I ordered my hot and sour soup from my neighborhood Chinese takeout, and took advantage of feeling good. Around 1:30 a.m., I took a sleeping pill and—lo and behold—I slept for a few hours, got up to pee from all the liquids I drank, and went back to bed. I rolled out around 8 a.m. and felt good. It was Friday, June 1 and, if I continued to feel good, I would go out to breakfast, do some banking, go to a movie, and maybe have dinner with the guys. It was 10 a.m., and off I went.

It was a pretty good day. I accomplished what I set out to do. The movie was good, and I got home in time to relax and do some things around the house. I slept alright with the pill, but I still got up to pee and take a swig of water to keep my mouth moist. I was waiting for the other shoe to drop, and it usually did around the third day. So Saturday should be okay, but Sunday might be a different story.

I got up out of bed at 8 a.m., and felt pretty good. I planned on going out for breakfast and reading my paper, and then doing some banking. The rest of the day had no plans in it. If someone called me for dinner, I would probably be able to go.

I was also doing a lot of thinking about this great big "Celebration of Life" party that I was planning for November. With my daughter-in-law catering it, this party would be one that people would talk about for a long while. Parties were much more fun than funerals. I have lost many people close to me, so I knew the difference. I loved parties, and this one would be my best one yet.

It was June 2, and I could see the light at the end of my tunnel. The rest of the day was fine. I actually spent about five hours sitting with my pregnant daughter, who was due the next week. It was good seeing her, as I didn't know when I would feel good enough to take the ride to see my new grandchild.

I went to sleep, or tried to go to sleep, around 1 a.m. It was another rough night, even with the pill. I did not get out of bed on Sunday until 11 a.m., and knew the other shoe had dropped. The garbage taste was back in my mouth, and it remained there no matter what I ate or drank. My tiredness returned, as my legs felt like Jell-O. So I was going to dig in for the next few weeks, knowing that when I started to feel better, it would continue, and I was getting no more of that poison in my system. I was ready for the fatigue.

I had a hard time, as usual, in falling asleep last night. This horrific taste in my mouth still existed. Today, I was going to the grocery store to look for sugar-free ice cream. Maybe, just maybe, that would help. For dinner, I would have hot and sour soup, which seemed to be spicy enough to make a dent in the bad taste.

I would also journey out to the post office and then to breakfast. By that time, my strength would be about all used up. It was Monday, June 4, four days after my last treatment.

Last night was a little better, as the ice cream seemed to help out a little. Around 12:30 a.m., I had an idea. I went down to the kitchen and made a peanut butter sandwich, which helped. I could not tell you why, but maybe I found the secret.

My sleep night was the usual. Tossed and turned, got up to pee, and finally fell asleep around 5:30 a.m. I opened my eyes at 9 a.m. and just stayed in bed until 11 a.m. I went out to breakfast and came back to watch a movie in my theater.

Hopefully I'd feel good enough to join a friend for dinner. I'd see how today went; one never knows.

And I also now experienced pain down by my legs, especially in my joints. Not a sharp pain, but something that let me know it was there. I'd had this side effect before, but it did not usually last. So I was thinking this would not last long either.

It was noon on Wednesday, June 6, and I was just rolling out of bed. I had the most horrible night yet. The pain in my legs was so persistent that I could scream. I never thought that it could get that bad. The bad taste had lightened up a little, but it would probably be back. I felt like I'd hit the wall.

Today I would not venture out of the house. Instead, I put myself in my most comfortable spot in my man cave, where I watched movies. Another night like I just had would be unbearable.

So I spent the better part of the day in the basement. I came up for dinner, even though I was not hungry and nothing seemed to kill this bad taste in my mouth.

I went into my bedroom at 10:30 p.m. I took three Advil and two Tylenol PM, which was what my nurse advised, and hoped for the best.

CHAPTER 17

WEEK ELEVEN

Today was Thursday, June 7, and after taking what my nurse advised me to, I actually fell asleep at 11 p.m. last night and opened my eyes at 5 a.m. That was huge, as I had not had that much straight sleep in a long time. I did not get up to pee, and was not disturbed by joint pain. I still had that crude taste in my mouth but, overall, I'd gotten some rest.

I stayed in bed until 10 a.m., and it felt good. I had nothing planned for the day except opening my front door and picking up my newspaper. I was not hungry, just thirsty, so I just drank to stay hydrated.

My daughter was dropping off some more Advil for me so I don't have to go out, as my legs were like rubber. Some new movies were delivered to me in the mail yesterday, so I would go into the cave and watch them. I seemed to be most comfortable in the man cave, as it was dark and the couch was soft. I was praying that each day would be better than the previous one.

That night was similar to the previous night, as I took my pills and slept. It was 11:30 p.m. when I fell asleep, and I opened my eyes at 5:30 a.m. I did notice something that was very important. The bad taste was dissipating, which was a major thing. The bad taste was the first thing that would leave me in my recovery.

I did not have to drink in the middle of the night, which was a first. But I was really tired and could not get out of bed. I just stayed there and fell asleep, and finally rolled out at noon. I still had minimal knee and ankle pain, but could live with that.

This day was half over, which I liked, as I wanted to push the time away. I had nothing planned but my usual day. I was really hoping to have a good weekend, not that I had any plans.

I spent most of the day in my basement in my favorite position, which I am sure anyone could figure out. About 5 p.m., I went upstairs to figure out what I wanted to eat for dinner. I did not eat all day, as I was not the slightest bit hungry. I decided on a frozen pizza, since I could finally taste it.

After dinner, I headed up to watch the ballgame in my favorite position. I seemed to be quite comfortable watching TV in my second bedroom, lying on the bed. It was now 10:30 p.m., and I would get ready for bed and watch TV after I took my pills. I really hoped to have a little more energy back tomorrow, and to get up before noon. We would see.

———

Not a bad night last night. I slept pretty well, and got out of bed at 10:30 a.m. I seemed to have a little more energy today, and would attempt to go out to breakfast. I hadn't been out of the house for a few days, so that would be nice.

I was told that once I started to feel better, it would continue and each day would be better. I really didn't believe that I could go through this again. I knew that I was a strong person, but it was ridiculous what I felt like the other day. So I was looking forward to having a decent day today, and each day being better. This poison that was in my body really took its toll on me. I felt for everyone who has had to go through this ordeal.

It was Saturday, June 9, and nine days after my last treatment. What a difference a day, or a few days, could make.

———

I had another good night's sleep. I opened my eyes around 9:30 a.m., and just stayed in bed until 10:30 a.m., when I decided to get up. I really didn't know how I would feel until I put my feet on the floor and started walking. It appeared that all my energy arrived in the morning and, as the day went on, slowly left me. One day it would not, and when I felt really good I would continue to feel good. I had been doing a lot of thinking, and I decided that, if this cancer came back, I would not go through this again and instead call it a wrap. I could not conceive of myself having to do this again. My quality of life during this time was horrible.

There was a movie that I really want to see and, if I felt good in the afternoon, I would attempt to go see it. But if not, there was always tomorrow or the next day. It was Sunday, and I did like reading the Sunday papers. So I went out to take them off the front lawn and start my day.

It was a good Sunday, as I went to see a movie around 3:30 p.m. It ended about 6 p.m., and then I went to Potbelly's, as I had a craving for a meatball sandwich. I just wished I could taste it. I had ordered my sandwich, a bag of chips, and a pickle. I sat outside and ate my dinner while enjoying a beautiful evening.

To show how my appetite had changed, I ate half the pickle, half the bag of chips, left some of my sandwich, and was quite satisfied. I just did not have an appetite. Maybe for me that was a good thing, as I could stand to lose ten pounds. Normally I would have lost weight, but the steroids in my system worked against me.

I wanted to take in the beautiful evening and just sit and watch people. The next thing I knew, it was 8 p.m. and I'd been sitting for two hours. I was starting to get tired, so I headed for my car and drove home, which took about three minutes.

I watched TV for a few hours, then decided to turn off the lights and TV and try to fall asleep. I was sleeping pretty well by now and, when I got up in the morning at whatever time I chose, I did feel rested.

On Monday, June 11, I was going to the post office to mail some letters, and then to lunch. At night, a friend was taking me to dinner, which I was looking forward to.

I rested most of the day, anticipating my dinner with friends. I was picked up around 6 p.m., as we had reservations at 6:15 p.m. Dinner for me was a waste, as I could not taste my skirt steak or sweet potato. I could not wait until I got some taste buds back. We had a good conversation and did not leave until around 8 p.m.

My friend is a cancer survivor and he told me like it was. He said the fourth round was so terrible that anybody who had not had it would never understand. He said it would take a while for my body to heal from all the poison.

When I got home, I was really tired. So tired that it took me a few minutes to walk up the stairs. I ran out of breath and had to sit down. I was looking forward to going into my bed and getting comfortable. I prayed that my decent nights of sleep continued.

It took a long time to fall asleep last night. I tried without taking pills, but that was stupid on my part. Tonight I would go back to my routine, as sleep was very important in getting my body back in shape.

It was 10 a.m. and I was not sure how I felt yet. I had no plans, and would spend the afternoon watching movies in the basement. I was not hungry and did not know what I would eat. I wished coffee didn't have to taste like mud.

So today was Tuesday, June 12. It had been twelve days since my last treatment, and I was wondering when I would start to feel better.

The day wound up being a total waste. I was really fatigued, and ran out of breath with the slightest thing that I did. I was ready for sleep, and hoped that I could get some. Maybe tomorrow I would feel a pinch better. We would see.

I had a decent night's sleep, but still felt very weak. I ran out of breath no matter what I did, even just brushing my teeth or walking from room to room. This was something I did not have during my previous three rounds of chemo. I was still in that three-week period, so I hoped it would just go away soon.

I was supposed to go to my high school the next day for an end-of-the-year party, so today I would just do nothing but relax. Relaxing seemed to be the thing that I did best. I had no appetite and did not believe I even had anything in the house to eat, but I did have liquids to drink.

I would probably order out for dinner and forgo lunch, as I regularly ate only two meals a day. Now it seemed like it had become one meal a day. The day was just starting, and I was hoping for a feel-good day.

Wishful thinking. I was really sick today. I called my nurse and made an appointment to see the doctor tomorrow. I had a hard time breathing. My kids were so worried about me that they insisted that someone stay with me, and I could not fight them.

I did not feel well, and hoped what I had was nothing really serious, where I would have to be hospitalized. Honestly, I just hoped to live through the night.

That evening I went out to dinner with a couple of my friends. I was not feeling too well, as I had a tough time catching my breath. My friends commented on how bad I looked.

After dinner, I went home and seemed to get even sicker. I spoke with my children, and they were so concerned that my daughter-in-law drove in from Milwaukee to spend the night with me. She took my temperature when she arrived. When it showed 100.5 degrees, she insisted that we go to the emergency room.

So off we went, as I did not object and could hardly catch my breath. I was starting to get scared. What I was experiencing was not good.

When we arrived, the emergency room was crowded, but they took me right in as I was having a tough time breathing. They did an EKG and a chest X-ray on me, which showed that my upper lungs were cloudy. That meant pneumonia, so I was going to be admitted.

CHAPTER 18

WEEK TWELVE

It was after midnight when I was finally assigned a room. My port was accessed, and I was hooked up to the IV machines. Every ten minutes or so, someone came into my room to ask the same questions. It was around 2:30 a.m., and I sent my daughter-in-law to sleep at my house, as I did not want her sleeping at the hospital.

It was Thursday, June 14, and I was about to spend five nights in the hospital.

The first night, I got zero sleep. I thought enough blood was taken from me to start another person. I met with several interns, a lung doctor, a cardiologist, and an infectious-disease doctor. Their job was to figure out what I actually had, and how to treat it.

I knew that, as long as I was in the hospital, sleep was not in the program for me. I would ask for a sleeping pill, but that didn't seem to work on me.

I was a little nervous, as I ran out of breath after I took two steps. I felt so bad that my mind had me thinking that I would not make it out of this alive.

I was told that what I was experiencing could be related to the chemo, which was my thought all along. Chemo-induced pneumonia had caused many people to be hospitalized. But first, the doctors had to rule out everything else, so they did a series of tests.

I must say that the nurses were absolutely great. They were nice, and answered every question that they could. And I had many questions.

I was on the eighth floor, which was the oncology floor. Not the best floor to be on but, since I had breast cancer, there was no other choice.

Every morning around 5:30 a.m., someone would come into my room to check my blood pressure and oxygen levels, and to take my blood. Forget any chance of sleep.

I was taken for a CT scan, which showed inflammation in my lungs. The question was what had caused this. Did I just get an infection from a weak immune system? Was this caused by chemo? Whatever caused this was making me really sick. I would get off the bed, take two steps, and be completely out of breath.

This feeling lasted until Friday. The doctors told me that I was anemic, and gave me two units of blood. For some reason, I felt a little better. I actually got off my bed and walked around a little bit.

The lung doctor came to see me, and it was decided that I'd be given some heavy-duty steroids. This was to clear up the inflammation in my chest.

A resident came to see me, and told me that they wanted to do a test to make sure that I had no acid in my blood. I asked him if it was painful, and he told me it was. I just didn't like pain, and this test required drawing blood from my wrist. The draw took about five minutes, and he was right—it was very painful. I just wanted to punch him in the nose.

Saturday turned out to be the day that I saved my life. Seeing that I was a borderline diabetic, I changed my menu to a diabetic one. When you had a diabetic menu, they automatically took your blood sugar before every meal. I knew that steroids drove blood sugars up, and I wanted to make sure that it was watched.

When they started taking my readings, they were off the chart. The machine that read the counts read them as high critical. They stuck my finger repeatedly, and each time it read the same. This was not good.

All food was cancelled from me and, at about 9 p.m. on Saturday, it was decided that I should be put in the intensive care unit so I could be watched very closely. On the ICU floor, each patient had one nurse. I found out that my blood sugars were at 602, which was quite frightening. I was given an insulin drip in my IV and, every hour on the hour, my nurse would prick my finger and get a reading.

Finally, my count started to drop. By 9 a.m. on Sunday, I was sent back to the eighth floor. My sugars were being managed, though they were still rather high.

I was starting to get some energy because of the steroids though, as long as I was on the steroids, my blood sugars would continue to be high. I was given a regular dose of insulin to keep the high blood sugars under some kind of control.

My lungs were clearing up, and I was given a breathing treatment three times a day by the respiratory department. I also began walking the halls, as I was feeling better and getting bored.

The insulin shots given to me were painless. I was told that, as long as I was taking the steroids, I would have the problem of higher blood sugars. I was also told that I was being weaned off the steroids, as stopping them cold turkey could cause damage.

By Monday, I was feeling much better, but was still quite weak. It was very hard to bounce back from pneumonia. It would take time to build up my endurance and get back to my normal routine. Plus I was getting the chemo out of my body.

My doctor came in to see me, and told me that he was sending me home on Tuesday. I was feeling good and walking the halls. I must say that not many people could walk the halls.

One thing that I did not mention. The night that I went into the hospital, I dropped my cell phone into the washing machine. I was phoneless, and all my contacts were washed away. So my daughter-in-law went to Verizon to pick me up a rental phone and order me another iPhone. I felt so helpless without a phone. No one knew that I was in the hospital.

My blood sugars were still high, and would remain that way until I was off the steroids. I was visited by a diabetes nurse and a nutritionist, and received an education from both. I was being sent home with a machine that would check my blood sugars. The little machine was covered by Medicare, and I was supposed to check my sugars before every meal and at bedtime, and chart the results.

I was also going to be sent home with steroid pills, which would gradually be cut back. The part that kind of shook me up was that I was also being sent home with insulin shots. I was put on a program where I would give myself insulin shots, with the amount determined by how high my count was. I had to be very careful not to administer more than I needed, for fear of falling blood sugars. That would cause a major problem.

On my last day, I was giving myself the shots under the nurse's supervision. The shots, I must say, were painless. I was so ready to go home. I was starting to get an appetite back, and the hospital meals were like eating dog food.

My discharge papers were like an instruction manual. I was given a bunch of prescriptions to be filled at the pharmacy, including pills, insulin pens, and needles to prick my finger.

It was around noon on Tuesday, June 19, when my friend picked me up to go home. Five hard days but, in the end, I was getting better and there was no more chemo to knock me back on my ass.

We stopped at the pharmacy, so I could get my meds and insulin pens. When I got home, I set up all my meds on a counter in an organized manner.

It was a little strange checking my blood sugars at first, using the special little pen with a needle that would prick my finger and draw the little blood that was needed to check my numbers. In time, doing it would become second nature.

My numbers were high, but I was not alarmed, as I was told they would be high and to just put the numbers in the book that I would give my doctor to check.

I was given a follow-up appointment on Thursday to see my doctor. That was two days away, and by that time I should be feeling even better.

It felt great to sleep in my own bed. I actually did get to sleep, and could sleep on my side or stomach. In a hospital bed, I'd had to sleep on my back, as the beds were so narrow and uncomfortable.

On Wednesday, it was really hot out, so I took in a movie after lunch. It was a little different eating three meals a day when I was used to eating only two, so I had to arrange my schedule to get up earlier, take my count, and then eat breakfast.

I was feeling stronger, and this was about the time that I was supposed to start feeling good again after chemo. In the past, I would then get zapped again and start to feel crappy. But now I would start to feel better each day and, in the next month or so, I would see my hair start to grow. I could see myself sitting in front of the mirror, watching my hair return.

On Thursday, I went to my follow-up appointment to see my doctor. He told me that I had a chemical pneumonia caused by the chemo. He told me that Friday would be my last day of the steroids. My blood sugars should then start to regulate, and I was to call him next week with my counts. I was also to cut down on my insulin, and eventually stop it altogether. I was to see him in two weeks and, at that time, he would tell me when I could have my port taken out.

This has been a really tough journey. I feel for anyone who has gone through chemo, or will have to go through it. You cannot know what it is like unless you have had to experience it.

I will probably be on tamoxifen for five years, and see the doctor every three months to be checked. I do know that I have a 89 percent chance of survival. Without the chemo, my chances would have been only 65 percent.

I like my new odds.

It is Friday, June 22, and I am on my way to start living my life again.

ABOUT THE AUTHOR

Richard W. Wiener is a retired high school teacher and athletic director. He has two children and three grandchildren, and resides in Glenview, Illinois.

He is a die-hard Chicago Blackhawks fan and, during hockey season, can be found at the United Center. He is also a member of the Chicago Public League Basketball Coaches Association Hall Of Fame.

He is also the author of "Check Please ... & Hurry," a book about dates gone wrong, which is already available. You can also find him at www.richwiener.com.

CPSIA information can be obtained at www.ICGtesting.com
Printed in the USA
LVOW08s0313130713

342609LV00003B/104/P